FIFTEEN SIMPLE MEATLESS RECIPES

To Share with Family and Friends

Natasha Ross

Fifteen Simple Meatless Recipes

Printed in the United States of America

First Printing, 2010

ISBN 978-1-387-03989-0

Atlanta, GA

Fifteen Simple Meatless Recipes

Fifteen Simple Meatless Recipes

CONTENTS

Fifteen Simple Meatless Recipes

Some of my family favorite recipes.

Natasha Ross

Make them your own by adding other things that you and your family enjoy.

My mother never used measurements when cooking and every one of her meal came out perfect.

Fifteen Simple Meatless Recipes

Macaroni & Cheese For Kids.

Ingredients.

- Macaroni

- Salt

- 1 cup of Shredded Parmesan cheese

- 1/2 cup Butter

- 1 1/2 cup sharp cheddar

- 1 cup Mozzarella cheese

- 3 1/2 cups of Milk

- 1/2 cup quinoa flour

- Sour cream

Directions.

1. Bring 4 cups of water to a boil with salt add macaroni cook for and drain macaroni preheat your oven to 275 degrees

2. 1 cup of Shredded Parmesan cheese 1/2 cup Butter 1 1/2 cup sharp cheddar 1 cup Mozzarella cheese 3 1/2 cups of Milk 1/2 cup quinoa flour Sour cream Bring 4 cups of water to a boil with salt add macaroni cook for and drain macaroni preheat your oven to 275 degrees In a large pot add butter flour and whisk on medium heat add milk and cheese continue to whisk add the macaroni to the mixture now add your sour cream and mix well. Put in a greased baking dish top with some shredded cheese and little more milk and bake for 30 to 40 minutes. Cool and serve My Granddaughter love it when I make this for her.

3. In a large pot add butter flour and whisk on medium heat add milk and cheese continue to whisk add the macaroni to the mixture and mix well.

4. Put in a greased baking dish top with some shredded cheese and little more milk and bake for 30 to 40 minutes.

5. Cool and serve.

My Granddaughter loves it when I make this for her. You may add eggs, I don't because she is allergic to eggs.

Tofu & Sour Cream Wrap.

Ingredients.

- 16 ounce package of tofu drain and cut into cubes
- 1 tbs. of butter
- 1 head of romaine lettuce
- 1 cup of shredded carrots
- 1 onion sliced
- 1/4 tbsp. of freshly chopped chives
- 1/2 tsp of oregano
- 2 diced garlic cloves
- 1 tsp red chili paste
- Sesame seeds
- Sour cream

Directions.

1. Put butter in pan on medium heat add garlic, onions and carrots, chopped ginger chili paste, oregano along with sesame seeds, stir for one minute on medium low heat then add tofu cook until tofu is slightly brown then add soy sauce and maple syrup cook for 2 additional mins and remove from heat.

Assembling of the wrap

2. I like to warm my tortilla on a griddle on each side for a few seconds.

3. I then place a lettuce leaf on each tortilla add some tofu and a dollop of sour cream then wrap and serve. You make the wrap to your desire there is no right or wrong way to enjoy them.

Tofu Salad With Mozzarella Cheese.

Ingredients.

- 12 ounce package of firm tofu

- 1 red onion sliced

- 24 cherry tomatoes cut into half

- One package of salad greens feel free to use freshly chopped greens as well

- 1 tsp of red wine vinegar

- Soy sauce

- Garlic

- 1/4 tsp of grated ginger

- 1 tbsp. of Asian chili sauce

Fifteen Simple Meatless Recipes

- Nonstick cooking spray

- 1/2 cup sliced black olives

- Shredded mozzarella cheese, as much as you want

Marinade For Tofu.

1. Drain and cut your tofu about 1 inch thick put the pieces into a bowl and add the soy sauce, minced ginger, Asian chili sauce, garlic, red wine vinegar for 30 minutes (longer if you like).

2. Remove from marinade don't discard the marinade save it to be used as the salad dressing. Now put your tofu onto the hot grill lightly sprayed with cooking spray cook on each side for 3 to 5 mins, cut tofu smaller when it cools.

Directions.

1. Put your green salad chopped, onions sliced, cherry tomatoes, sliced black olives and grilled tofu in a big salad bowl and toss with the left over Marinade.

2. Serve on salad plates and sprinkle with shredded mozzarella on the top.

Wild Rice With Fried Tofu & Veg.

Ingredients.

- 2 cups of wild rice

- 12 oz. packet of Tofu

- Onions

- Broccoli washed and cut

- Shredded carrots

- Salt and pepper

- Sesame oil

Directions For Wild Rice.

1. Rinse the wild rice under cold running water.

2. Bring 4 cups of water to a rolling boil.

3. Add wild rice, stir occasionally and cook on low heat until tender for 40-45 minutes and drain in colander.

Directions For Tofu.

1. Drain tofu cut into chunks in a mixing bowl.

2. Marinade tofu in soy sauce, minced ginger, chili sauce, garlic, rice wine vinegar for 30 minutes.

3. Remove from marinade save the marinade l. pat tofu dry and put into hot skillet with sesame oil and fry for 3mins on each side.

4. Put chopped broccoli.

5. And slice onions in the same skillet add broccoli and onions stir and add the tofu marinade and tofu cover for 3mins and serve over wild rice garnish with chopped Parsley.

Ziti Pasta Casserole With Portabella Mushrooms & Spinach.

Ingredients.

- 18 ounces of uncooked ziti pasta

- 1 cup of grated Parmesan cheese

- 1/2 cup mozzarella cheese

- 1 cup of chopped portabella mushrooms

- 1/2 cup chopped onions

- 10 ounce spinach of choice

- 1 red bell pepper chopped to desired size

Fifteen Simple Meatless Recipes

- 2 (24 oz.) jars of marinara sauce

- 1 cup of sour cream

- 1 tbsp. of olive oil Butter your of your choice

Directions.

1. Cook ziti pasta for 12 minutes in boiling water.

2. In a large pot add the pasta and all other ingredients and stir well.

3. Heat your oven to 350 degrees.

4. Lightly spray a 9-inch baking dish with nonstick cooking spray.

5. And pour ziti pasta mixture in the baking dish sprinkle the top with more parmesan cheese and bake for 35 to 40 minutes cheese will be nice and bubble.

Noodles With Grilled Tofu & Onions Sprinkled With Chives.

Ingredients.

- I packet of noodles

- 1pound packet of extra firm tofu

- Sea salt

- 2 garlic cloves minced

- 1/2 cup soy sauce

- 2 tbsp. of maple syrup (use sugar if you like)

- Red chili flakes to taste

- 2 onions washed and sliced

Fifteen Simple Meatless Recipes

- Sesame oil

- 1 tsp of freshly chopped ginger

Directions.

1. Bring a pot of water to a boil then add a package of noodles cook for 12 minutes.

2. Slice your tofu 1/2 an inch thick pat dry marinade in a bowl with salt and pepper ginger, soy sauce garlic sesame oil and red chili flakes for 15 minutes.

3. Heat your grill and spray with nonstick cooking spray. Save your marinade. Pat off the marinade with a paper towel before putting tofu on the grill, grill for 3 mins on each side.

4. Remove from grill and cut into chunks.

5. In a big put pour in a table spoon of sesame oil on medium heat add the grill chunks of tuff onions and noodle pour in the saved marinade and toss until the noodles is well coated add more soy sauce it needed. Serve hot and top with more onions if you desire.

Creamy Broccoli Florets Stuffed Pasta Shells.

Ingredients.

- 12 ounce box jumbo shells
- 2 cups of broccoli florets chopped
- Sea salt and fresh ground pepper
- 16 ounces of low-fat ricotta cheese
- 2 cup low-fat mozzarella cheese
- Half cup Parmesan cheese
- Chopped cilantro
- Chopped garlic
- Paprika
- Almond milk

Fifteen Simple Meatless Recipes

- Quinoa flour for thickening

Directions.

Cook the pasta shells for 10 mins.

Drain and put to cool on a baking.

Shell Stuffing Ingredients.

Mix 2 cups of broccoli florets chopped fresh ground pepper

16 ounces of low-fat ricotta cheese

2 cup low-fat mozzarella cheese

Sauce Ingredients.

- 3 tbsp. of butter

- 3 chopped garlic cloves

- 1 1/4 cup of almond milk

- 2 cup s of parmesan cheese

- 1/4 tsp of red pepper flakes

- Sea salt to taste

- Quinoa flour for thickening

- 2 tbsp. of chopped cilantro

- 2 tbsp. of chopped chives

- 1 cup of diced cherry tomatoes

Directions.

1. Take a 9×13 inch oven safe baking dish and spoon some of the sauce at the bottom then stuff the shells with the cheese and broccoli florets mixture now pour the remainder of the over the pasta shells sprinkle with chopped chives.

2. Put to bake for 35to 40 mins.

3. Cool serve enjoy with your family or friends.

Quinoa Dough Pizza With White Barbecue Sauce.

Ingredients For The Dough.

- 2 1/2 cups of quinoa flour

- 1/4 tsp of salt

- 1 1/2 tbsp. of avocado oil

- 1 tbsp. of maple syrup

- 1 cup of alkaline or spring water

Directions.

1. In a mixing bowl or dough maker.

2. Add quinoa flour, salt, oregano, maple syrup, avocado oil add the water slowly and mix to form a smooth dough.

3. Cover the dough for 40 mins to an hour.

Ingredients For The White Barbecue Sauce.

- 1 cup of Organic mayonnaise

- 4 garlic cloves finely chopped

- 1 tsp of horseradish

- 1/4 tsp of black pepper

- 1 tsp of maple syrup

- 1/3 of a tsp of Organic apple cider vinegar if you like but it can be left out

- 1/4 tsp of red pepper flakes

- 1/2 tsp of oregano

- Mix all of your ingredients together in a mixing bowl and refrigerate until you are ready for it.

Topping.

- 1 cup of Ricotta cheese

- 1 cup of shredded mozzarella cheese

- 1 red onion sliced to desire

- 1 yellow bell pepper washed and sliced

- Shiitake mushrooms washed and sliced

- 2 tbsp. fresh chopped scallions.

- A few fresh washed basil leaves

Directions.

1. Heat the oven 450 degrees F.

2. Lightly grease a 10 inch pizza tray.

3. Roll your quinoa dough on a floured surface until it is stretched to desired size to fit your pizza tray.

4. Add sauce and other toppings and bake for 10 minutes or until the edges are lightly brown cut your pizza and serve.

Spinach Fettuccine Squash & Tomato Recipe For Dinner.

Ingredients.

- 1 8oz ounce box of spinach fettuccine

- One yellow squash chopped

- 15 Cherry tomatoes chopped

- 2 tablespoons chopped chives

- 2 tablespoons chopped parsley

- Sea salt

- Hemp milk

- Red pepper flakes

Fifteen Simple Meatless Recipes

- Paprika

- 1/4 cup of butter

- 8 ounce Parmesan cheese

- 2 ounce plain cream cheese

Directions.

1. In a large pot add water and salt bring to boil for 12 to 15 minutes or according to directions on a box drain after fettuccine is cooked.

Ingredients & Directions For The Cream Sauce.

- In a saucepan over low heat add butter and garlic.

- Chop squash continue stirring.

- Next add chopped cherry tomatoes.

- Hemp milk.

- Parmesan cheese.

- Cream cheese continue stirring.

- Add paprika, black pepper, chopped parsley and chopped chives.

- We don't want any more salt because we already added salt to the fettuccine.

- Now add fettuccine to cream sauce toss and serve with a sprinkle of fresh parsley on the top and some red pepper flakes.

Garbanzo Bean Patties.

Ingredients.

- 2 cup of garbanzo bean flour
- Onions
- Mushrooms
- Bell pepper red
- Green bell pepper
- Cilantro
- Avocado oil or nonstick cooking spray
- Sea salt
- Thyme
- Basil
- Oregano
- Water

Fifteen Simple Meatless Recipes

Directions.

1. Chop the onions, mushrooms, red and green bell peppers small And cilantro place in a mixing bowl.

2. And add sea salt to taste, thyme, basil and oregano.

3. Add the garbanzo bean flour a little at a time and mix to a thick consistency.

4. Put your skillet to heat on medium and spray with nonstick cooking spray, use an ice cream scoop to scoop the mixture one at a time and drop into skillet cook on each side until golden brown

5. And serve with your favorite roll. You can also use a deep fryer or oil in the skillet.

Cucumber Salad With Chickpea.

Ingredients.

- 3 Cucumbers grated
- 1/4 tsp of sea salt
- 1 Onion finely diced
- I can of chickpea
- Black pepper
- 1/2 Lemon juice
- 2 tbsp. finely chopped parsley
- 1tbs dill
- 1/2 cup low-fat ricotta cheese
- 1 large red bell pepper roasted
- Red pepper flakes for a little spice

Directions.

1. Wash and grate your cucumbers and use a cheese cloth to squeeze out most of the liquid.

2. And onion, add to a big salad bowl.

3. Open can of chickpea and pour into a colander drain all of the liquid out

4. Now add chickpea to the cucumbers and onions, and add all other ingredients

5. Chop the roasted bell pepper and add to the dish lastly add the low-fat ricotta cheese and a sprinkle of red pepper flakes.

6. Serve with crackers or Bruschetta it can also be served as a side salad or on your favorite bread.

This is all about you and the way you will like to enjoy this recipe.

Cream Spinach Tortellini.

Ingredients.

- 1 packet of tortellini

- 1 packet of frozen spinach, fresh if you like

- 1 tbsp. of avocado oil

- 1/4 tsp of sea salt

- 1 tbsp. ground tarragon

- Scallions

- 2 garlic cloves finely chopped

- Black pepper to taste

- 1 1/2 cup of hemp milk

- 1/2 cup of grated parmesan cheese

- 1/2 cup of mozzarella cheese

- 1 tbsp. of Organic olive oil butter

Fifteen Simple Meatless Recipes

Directions.

1. In a pot bring 3 quarts of water to a boil add salt if you like and add the tortellini, let cook for 11 minutes be sure to stir I like to add a table spoon of oil so that my tortellini doesn't stick together.

2. In a big sauce pan add organic olive oil butter and garlic stir for 30 seconds now add your spinach and scallions, tarragon black pepper parsley.

3. Hemp milk or milk of choice.

4. Now add your cheeses.

5. And stir simmer on low heat.

6. Now drain tortellini and add it to your creamy spinach sauce

7. Toss to coat your tortellini very well

8. And serve with a sprinkle of parsley on the top.

Veg & Quinoa.

Ingredients.

- 2 Zucchini

- 1 grated carrot

- 2 Garlic cloves

- 1 onion

- Cilantro

- 2oz mushrooms

- 1 red bell pepper

- 1 green bell pepper

- 1yellow bell pepper

- Avocado oil

- Sea salt to taste

- Oregano

- Ground thyme

Directions.

1. Wash and Chop all ingredients into desired shapes.

2. Heat a large pan add avocado oil then chopped garlic.

3. Add all ingredients and stir in seasonings.

4. Cover for 3 mins.

5. Then add the mushrooms stir and cover for another 2 mins. Stir and remove from heat.

For the quinoa

6. Bring 4 cups of water to a boil add salt if you desire.

7. Put 3 cups of quinoa in a fine strainer and rinse quinoa with cold water.

8. Add quinoa to boiling water on medium heat and let cook until tender.

9. Drain in fine strainer.

10. And serve with vegetables.

Curry Mango Served With Wild Rice.

Ingredients.

- 3 green mangoes cut into pieces and washed

- 6 garlic cloves

- 2 tbsp. of avocado oil

- 1/4 tsp of salt

- 2 tbsp. of curry powder mix in 1/2 cup of water

- 1/2 maple syrup

- Black pepper if you desire

Directions.

1. Boil the chopped mangos for 20 mins then drain.

2. Mix the curry powder in a 1/2 of water and stir.

3. Heat a medium size source pan on medium heat, now add the oil and the chopped garlic. Now carefully pour in the curry powder in a 1/2 of water and stir for about 1 min.

4. Carefully add the chopped mangos.

5. Stir add salt and add one cup of water.

6. Add maple syrup stir and cover with lid and simmer on low for 40 to 45 minute.

7. Serve with wild rice.

Spinach Pasta With Mushrooms.

Ingredients.

- One box of spinach pasta 1 box of spinach pasta one box of spinach pasta, feel free to use any type of pasta you like

- Two ounce of mushrooms of your choice chopped

- One cup of hemp milk

- Use the milk of your choice

- 2 Bell peppers washed and chopped

- 1/2 tsp Sea salt

- 3 tbsp. of chopped Cilantro

- 1/3 of a tsp of paprika

- 1/2 cup of organic olive oil Butter

- Cheese

Directions.

1. Cook pasta until it's al dente or your desire and drain.

2. Add the Butter to the pan then add chopped mushrooms.

3. Bell peppers, cooked pasta, milk and cheese, salt to taste stir and add paprika and some cilantro stir and serve hot, garnish with a little more cilantro.

Acknowledgements.

I would like to express my love and appreciation to my family and friends, who has always been big supporters to me, although I didn't tell them about this book I know you all are very happy and excited.

Most importantly, I have to say thank you to my mom for teaching me how to cook!

Thank you to each and every one of you that has decided to try my meals.

www.ingramcontent.com/pod-product-compliance
Lightning Source LLC
Chambersburg PA
CBHW050342290526
45785CB00006B/2602